- Table of Conte

MW00953580

Internal Organs of Dog
Bones of Dog
Muscles of Dog
Arterial Circulatory System of Dog
Nerves of Dog
....
Internal Organs of Cat
Bones of Cat
Muscles of Cat
Arterial System of Cat
Nerves of Cat
....
Internal Organs of Horse
Bones of Horse
Muscles of Horse
Veins and Arteries of Horse
Nerves of Horse
....
Internal Organs of Frog
Bones of Frog
Muscles of Frog
Arteries and Veins of Frog
....
Internal Organs of Cow
Bones of Cow
Muscles of Cow
....
Internal Organs of Bird
Bones of Bird
Muscles of Bird
....
Internal Organs of Elephant
Bones of Elephant
Muscles of Elephant
....
Internal Organs of Dolphin
Bones of Dolphin
Muscles of Dolphin
....
Internal Organs of Deer
Bones of Deer
Muscles of Deer

Internal Organs of Zebra
Bones of Zebra
Muscles of Zebra
....
Internal Organs of Tiger
Bones of Tiger
Muscles of Tiger
....
Bones of Bear
Muscles of Bear
....
Bones of Hippo
Muscles of Hippo
....
Bones of Rhinoceros
Muscles of Rhinoceros
....
Bones of Wolf
Muscles of Wolf
....
Bones of Giraffe
Muscles of Giraffe
....
Bones of Camel
Muscles of Camel
....
Bones of Mountain Lion
Muscles of Mountain Lion
....
Bones of Red Kangaroo
Muscles of Red Kangaroo
....
Bones of Jack Rabbit
Muscles of Jack Rabbit
....
Internal Organs of Guinea Hen
Muscles of Guinea Hen
....
Internal Organs of Chicken
Bones of Chicken

Internal Organs of Dog

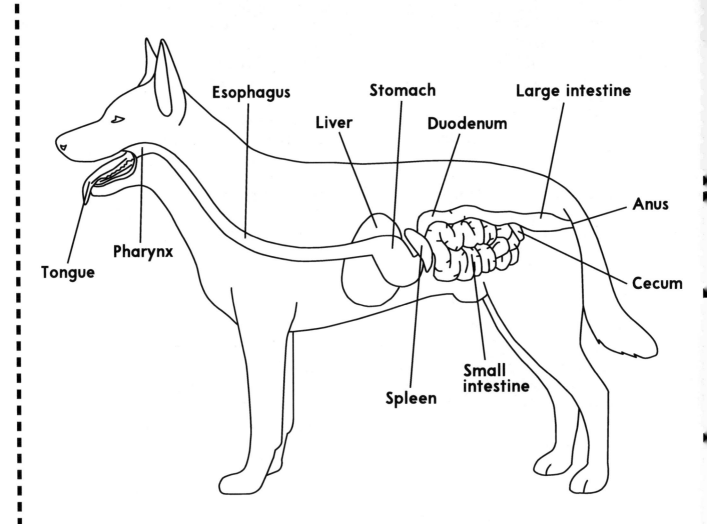

Bones of Dog

German Shepherd Dog

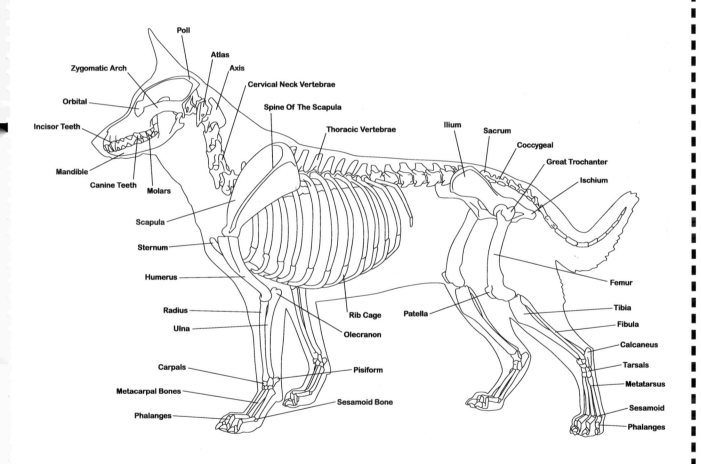

Muscles of Dog
German Shepherd Dog

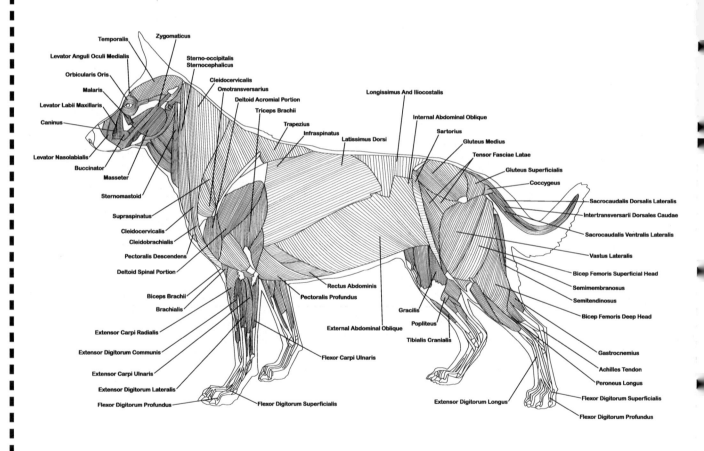

Arterial Circulatory System Of Dog

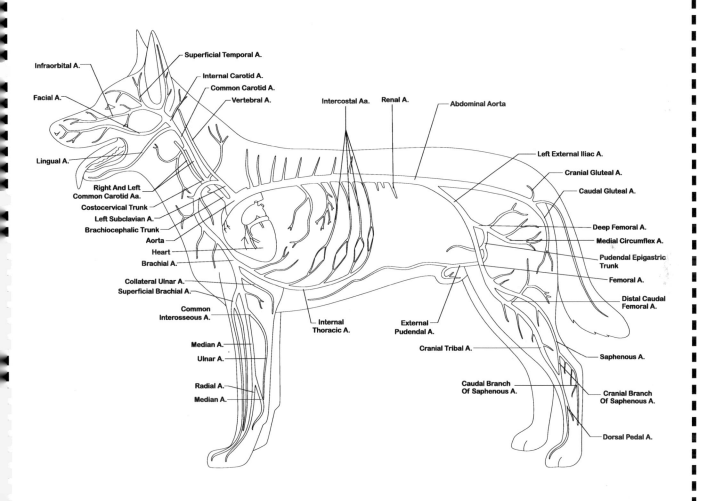

Superficial Temporal A.

Infraorbital A.

Internal Carotid A.

Common Carotid A.

Facial A.

Vertebral A.

Intercostal Aa.

Renal A.

Abdominal Aorta

Lingual A.

Left External Iliac A.

Cranial Gluteal A.

Caudal Gluteal A.

Right And Left
Common Carotid Aa.

Costocervical Trunk

Left Subclavian A.

Brachiocephalic Trunk

Deep Femoral A.

Medial Circumflex A.

Aorta

Pudendal Epigastric
Trunk

Heart

Brachial A.

Femoral A.

Collateral Ulnar A.

Superficial Brachial A.

Distal Caudal
Femoral A.

Common
Interosseous A.

Internal
Thoracic A.

External
Pudendal A.

Median A.

Cranial Tribal A.

Saphenous A.

Ulnar A.

Radial A.

Caudal Branch
Of Saphenous A.

Cranial Branch
Of Saphenous A.

Median A.

Dorsal Pedal A.

Nerves of Dog

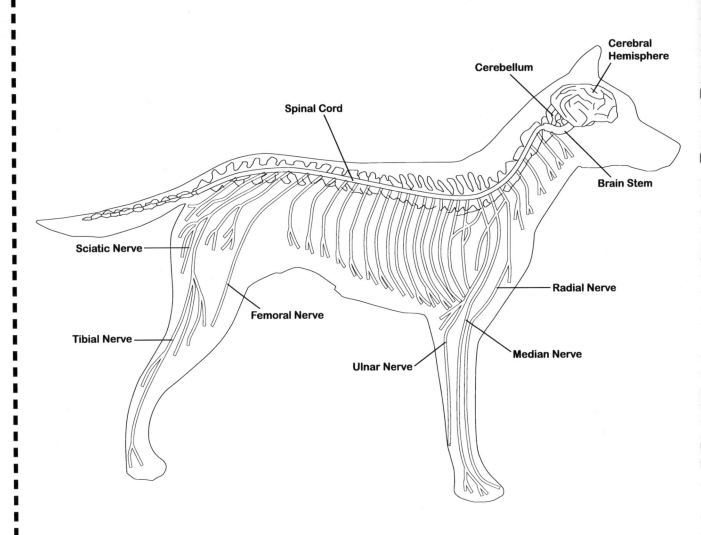

Internal Organs of Cat

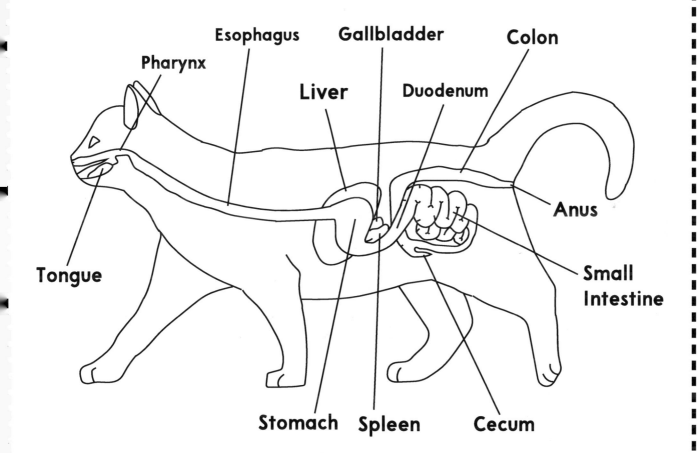

Bones of Cat

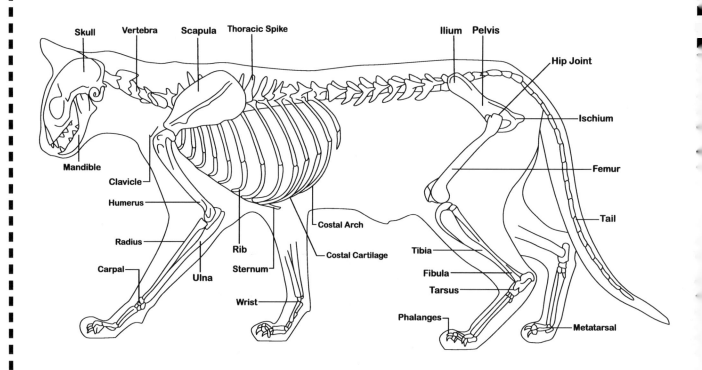

Muscles of Cat

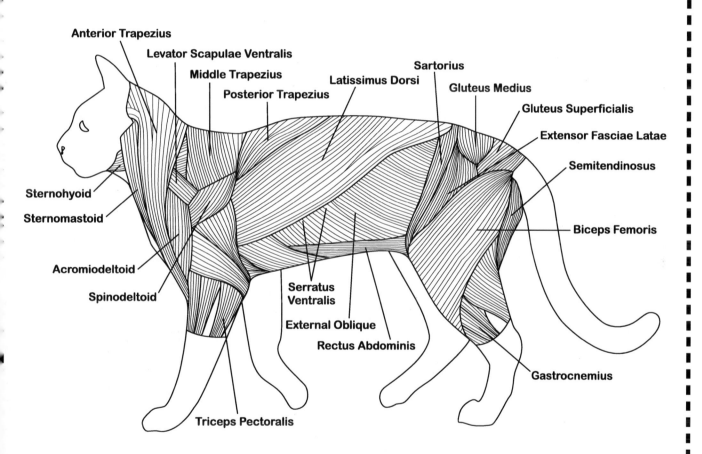

Arterial System Of The Cat

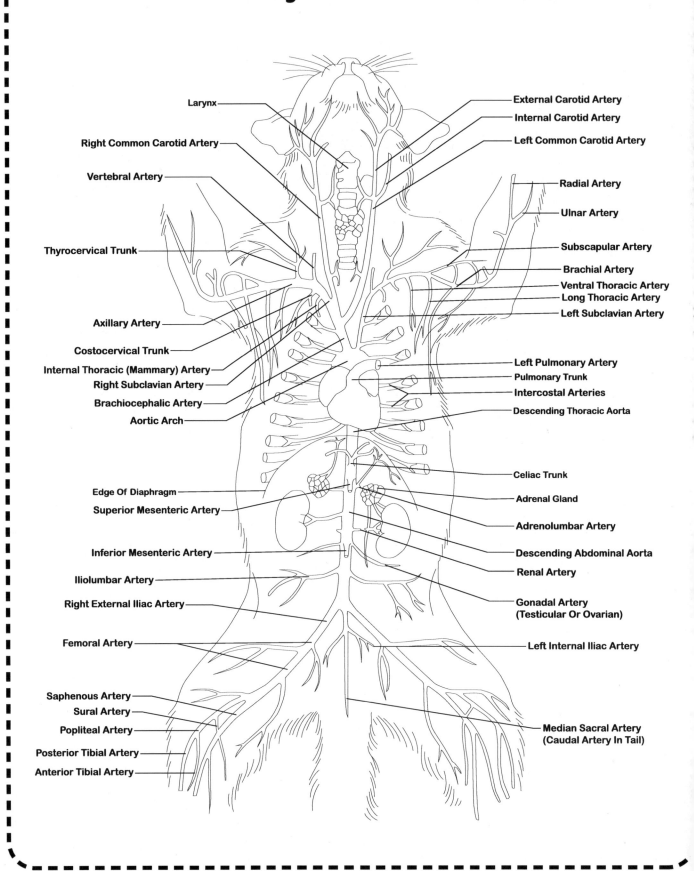

- Larynx
- Right Common Carotid Artery
- Vertebral Artery
- Thyrocervical Trunk
- Axillary Artery
- Costocervical Trunk
- Internal Thoracic (Mammary) Artery
- Right Subclavian Artery
- Brachiocephalic Artery
- Aortic Arch
- Edge Of Diaphragm
- Superior Mesenteric Artery
- Inferior Mesenteric Artery
- Iliolumbar Artery
- Right External Iliac Artery
- Femoral Artery
- Saphenous Artery
- Sural Artery
- Popliteal Artery
- Posterior Tibial Artery
- Anterior Tibial Artery

- External Carotid Artery
- Internal Carotid Artery
- Left Common Carotid Artery
- Radial Artery
- Ulnar Artery
- Subscapular Artery
- Brachial Artery
- Ventral Thoracic Artery
- Long Thoracic Artery
- Left Subclavian Artery
- Left Pulmonary Artery
- Pulmonary Trunk
- Intercostal Arteries
- Descending Thoracic Aorta
- Celiac Trunk
- Adrenal Gland
- Adrenolumbar Artery
- Descending Abdominal Aorta
- Renal Artery
- Gonadal Artery (Testicular Or Ovarian)
- Left Internal Iliac Artery
- Median Sacral Artery (Caudal Artery In Tail)

Nerves of Cat

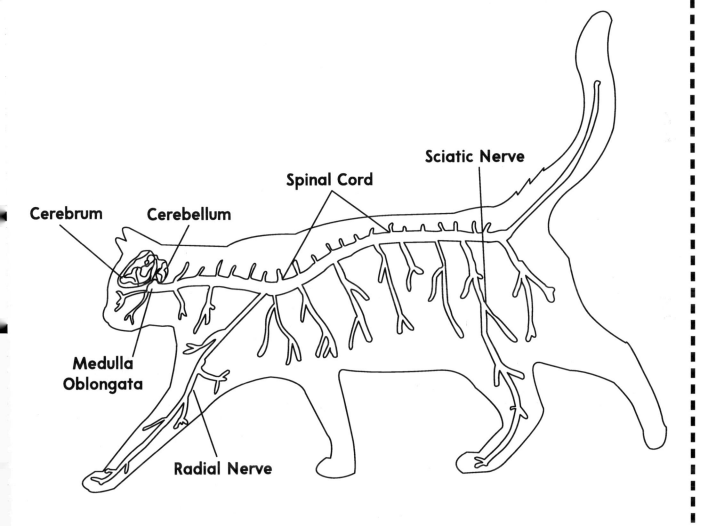

Cerebrum

Cerebellum

Spinal Cord

Sciatic Nerve

Medulla
Oblongata

Radial Nerve

Internal Organs of Horse

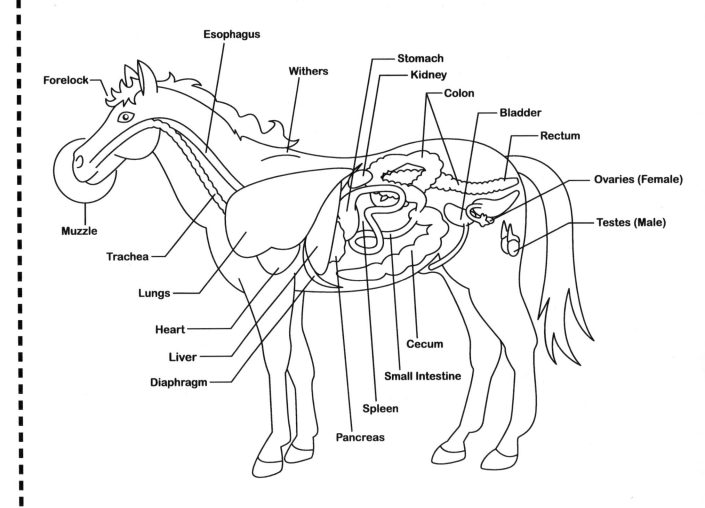

Bones of Horse

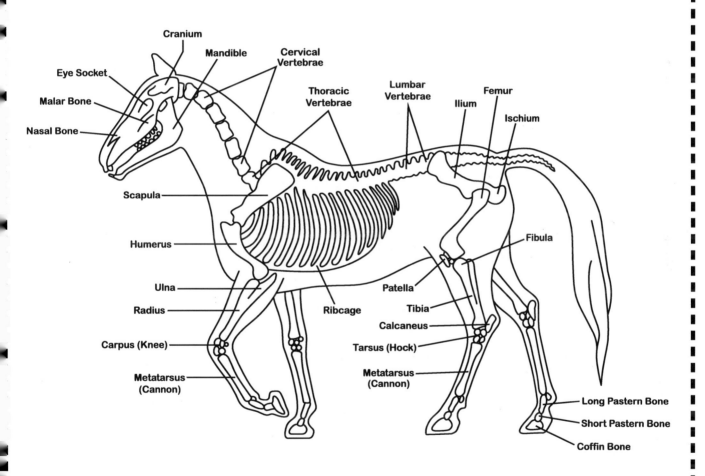

Muscles of Horse

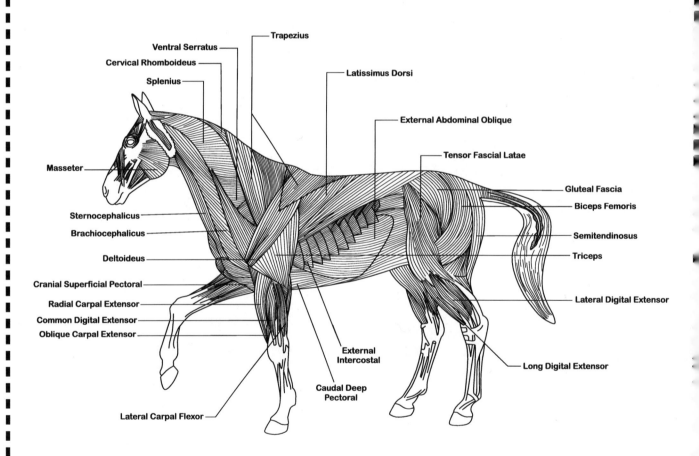

Veins And Arteries of Horse

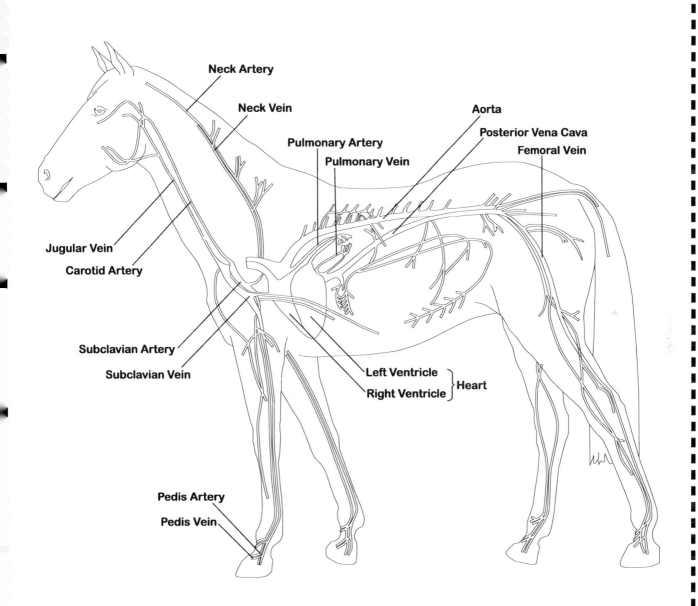

Nerves of Horse

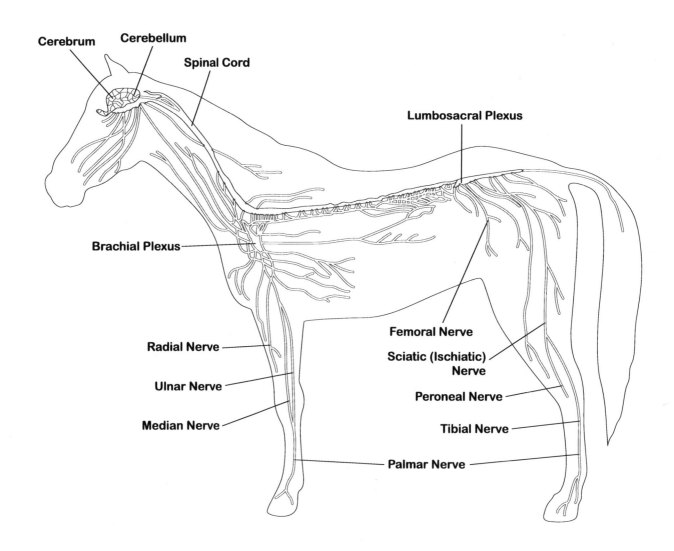

Cerebrum
Cerebellum
Spinal Cord
Lumbosacral Plexus
Brachial Plexus
Femoral Nerve
Sciatic (Ischiatic) Nerve
Radial Nerve
Ulnar Nerve
Peroneal Nerve
Median Nerve
Tibial Nerve
Palmar Nerve

Internal Organs of Frog

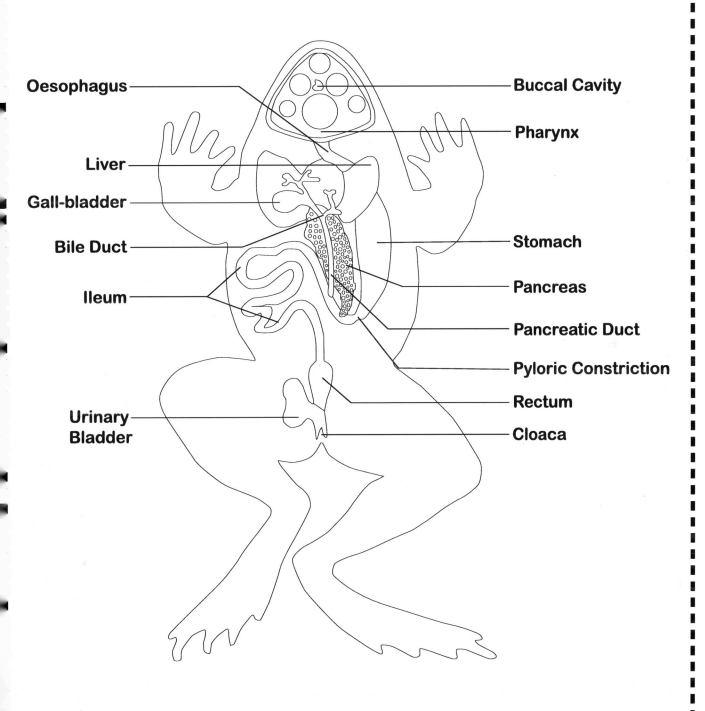

Oesophagus

Liver

Gall-bladder

Bile Duct

Ileum

Urinary
Bladder

Buccal Cavity

Pharynx

Stomach

Pancreas

Pancreatic Duct

Pyloric Constriction

Rectum

Cloaca

Bones of Frog

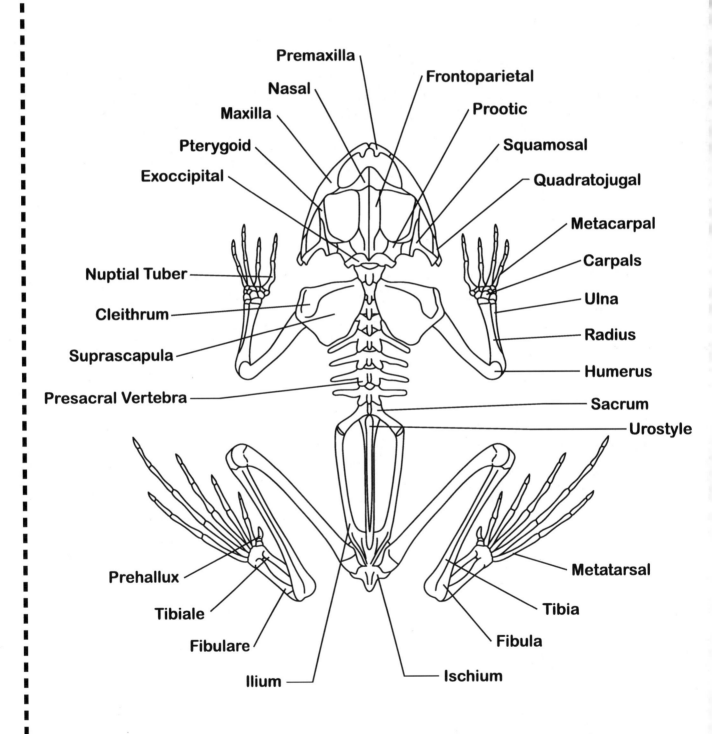

Muscles of Frog

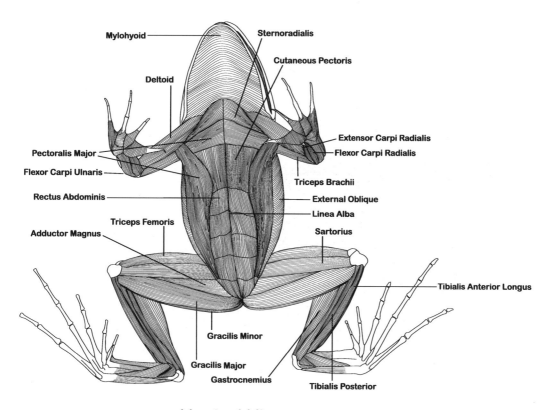

- Mylohyoid
- Sternoradialis
- Cutaneous Pectoris
- Deltoid
- Extensor Carpi Radialis
- Flexor Carpi Radialis
- Pectoralis Major
- Flexor Carpi Ulnaris
- Triceps Brachii
- Rectus Abdominis
- External Oblique
- Linea Alba
- Triceps Femoris
- Sartorius
- Adductor Magnus
- Tibialis Anterior Longus
- Gracilis Minor
- Gracilis Major
- Gastrocnemius
- Tibialis Posterior

Ventral View

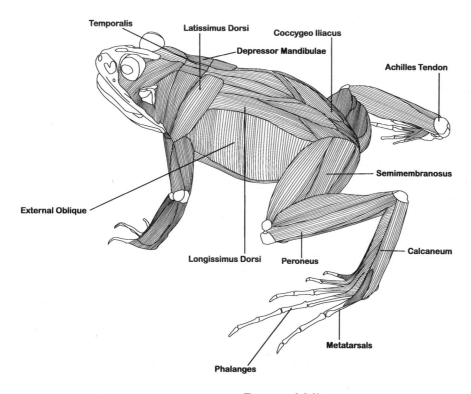

- Temporalis
- Latissimus Dorsi
- Coccygeo Iliacus
- Depressor Mandibulae
- Achilles Tendon
- Semimembranosus
- External Oblique
- Longissimus Dorsi
- Peroneus
- Calcaneum
- Metatarsals
- Phalanges

Dorsal View

Arteries and Veins of Frog

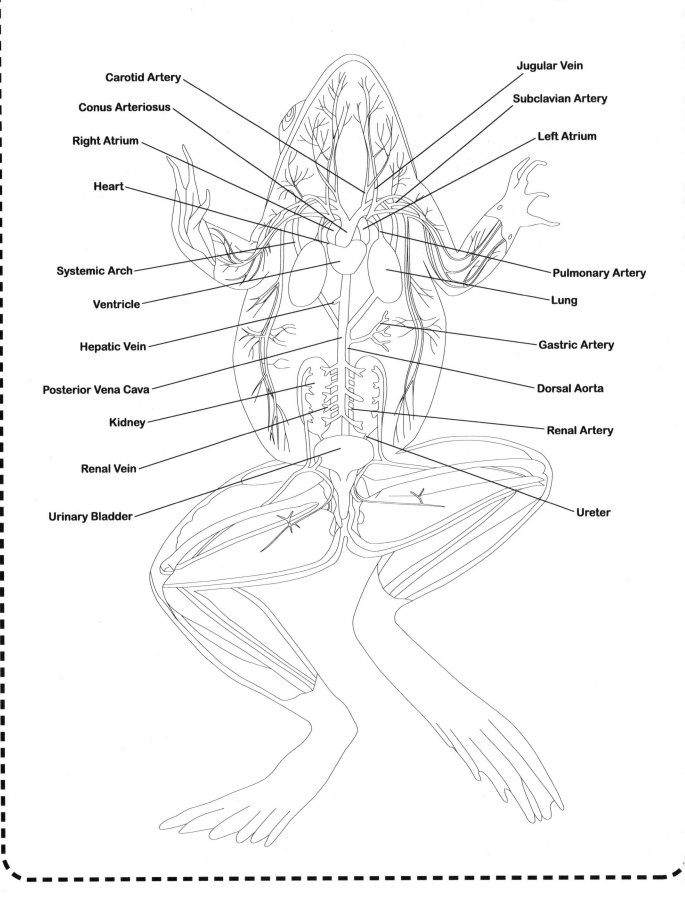

Carotid Artery

Conus Arteriosus

Right Atrium

Heart

Systemic Arch

Ventricle

Hepatic Vein

Posterior Vena Cava

Kidney

Renal Vein

Urinary Bladder

Jugular Vein

Subclavian Artery

Left Atrium

Pulmonary Artery

Lung

Gastric Artery

Dorsal Aorta

Renal Artery

Ureter

Internal Organs of Cow

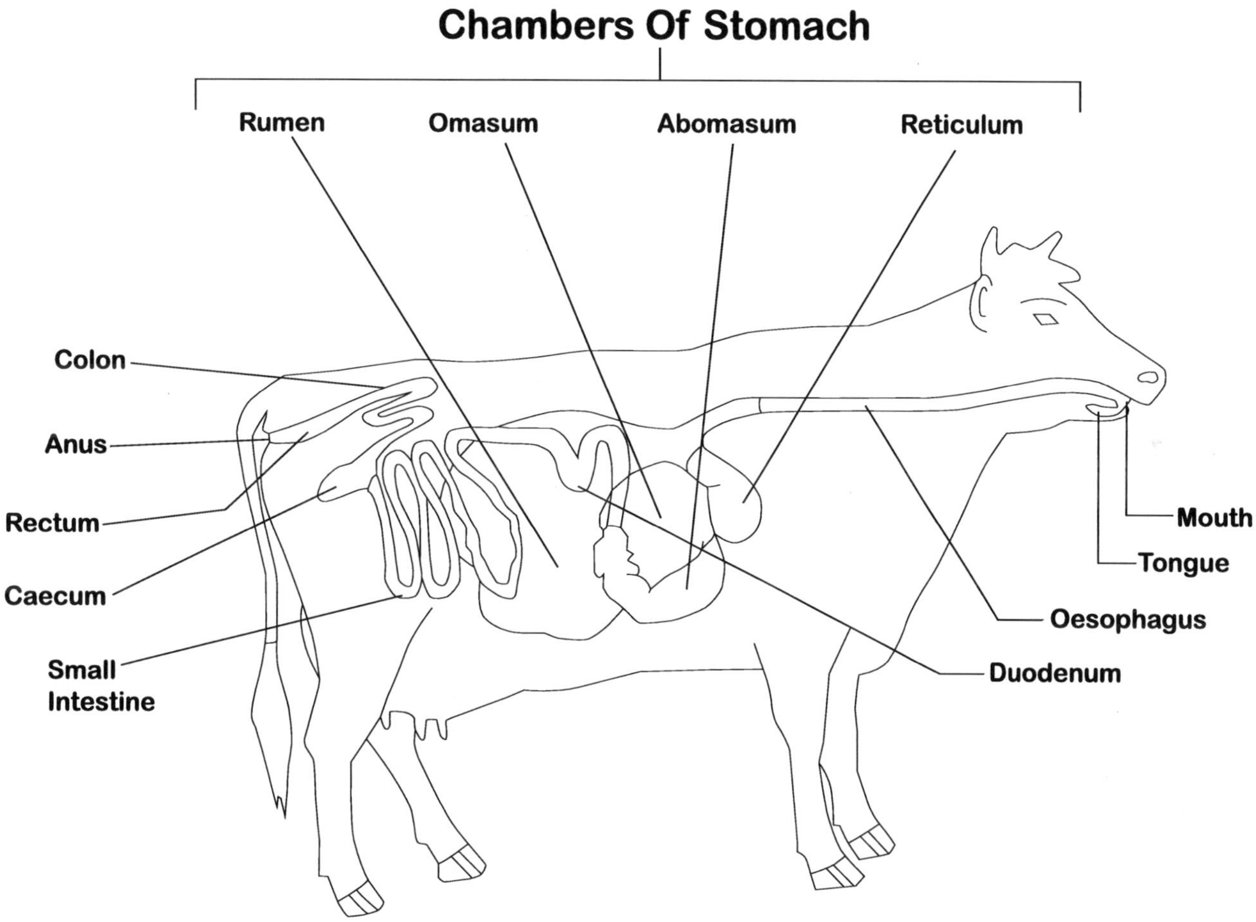

Chambers Of Stomach

Rumen   Omasum   Abomasum   Reticulum

Colon

Anus

Rectum

Caecum

Small
Intestine

Mouth

Tongue

Oesophagus

Duodenum

Bones of Cow

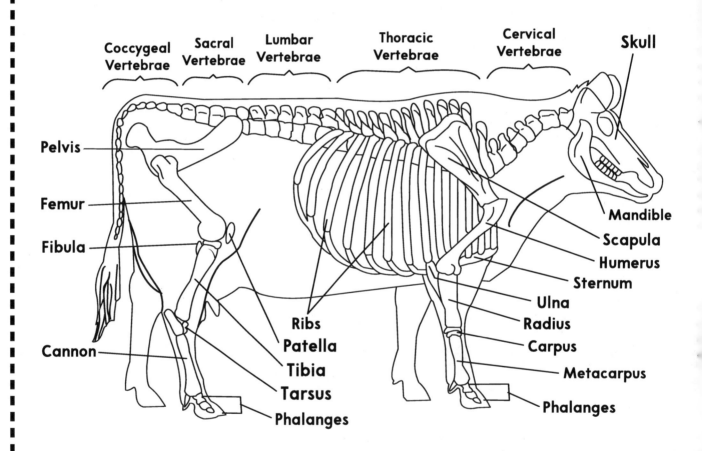

Coccygeal Vertebrae · Sacral Vertebrae · Lumbar Vertebrae · Thoracic Vertebrae · Cervical Vertebrae · Skull

Pelvis · Femur · Fibula · Cannon

Ribs · Patella · Tibia · Tarsus · Phalanges

Mandible · Scapula · Humerus · Sternum · Ulna · Radius · Carpus · Metacarpus · Phalanges

Muscles of Cow

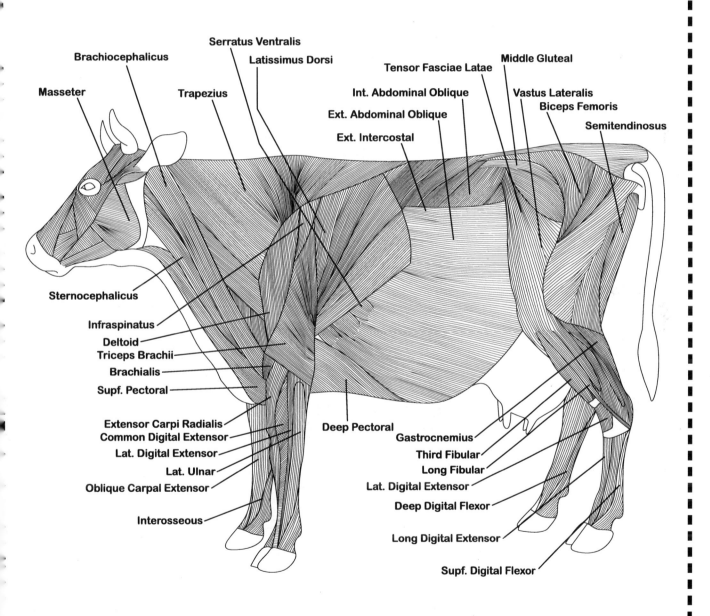

Brachiocephalicus

Serratus Ventralis

Latissimus Dorsi

Masseter

Trapezius

Tensor Fasciae Latae

Middle Gluteal

Int. Abdominal Oblique

Vastus Lateralis

Ext. Abdominal Oblique

Biceps Femoris

Ext. Intercostal

Semitendinosus

Sternocephalicus

Infraspinatus

Deltoid

Triceps Brachii

Brachialis

Supf. Pectoral

Extensor Carpi Radialis

Common Digital Extensor

Deep Pectoral

Gastrocnemius

Lat. Digital Extensor

Third Fibular

Lat. Ulnar

Long Fibular

Oblique Carpal Extensor

Lat. Digital Extensor

Deep Digital Flexor

Interosseous

Long Digital Extensor

Supf. Digital Flexor

Internal Organs of Bird

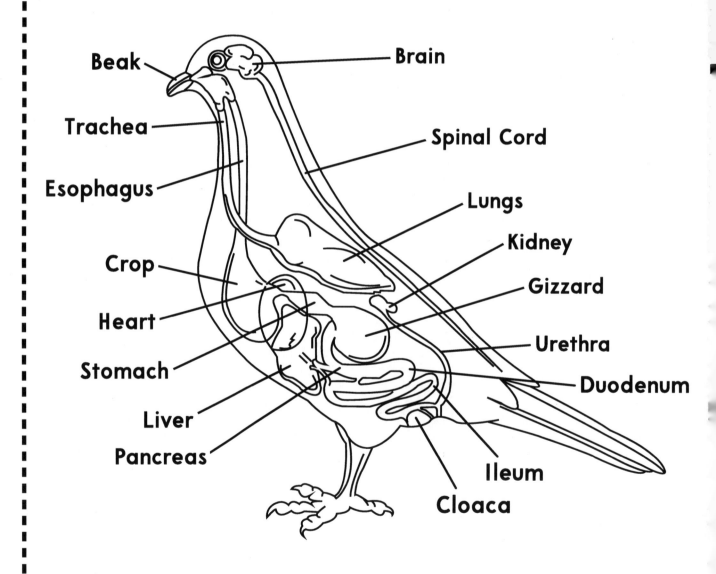

Beak

Trachea

Esophagus

Crop

Heart

Stomach

Liver

Pancreas

Brain

Spinal Cord

Lungs

Kidney

Gizzard

Urethra

Duodenum

Ileum

Cloaca

Bones of Bird

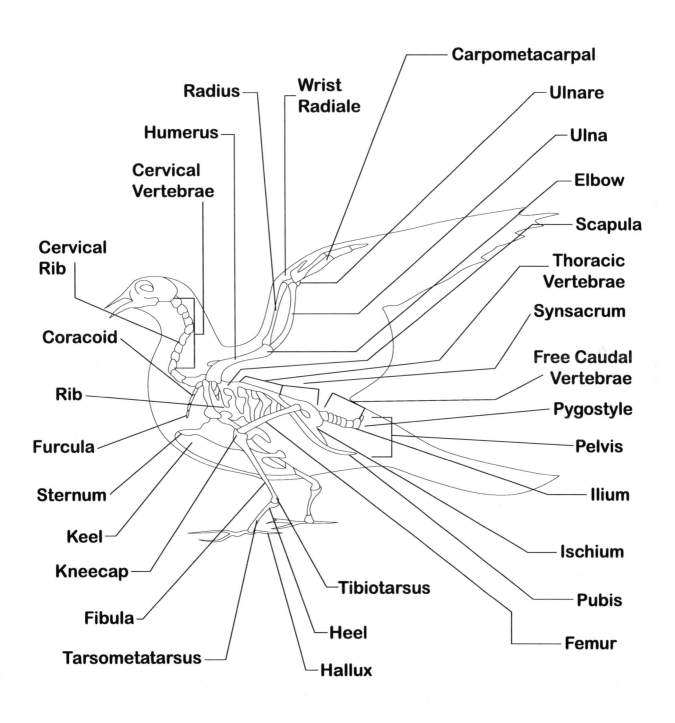

Muscles of Bird

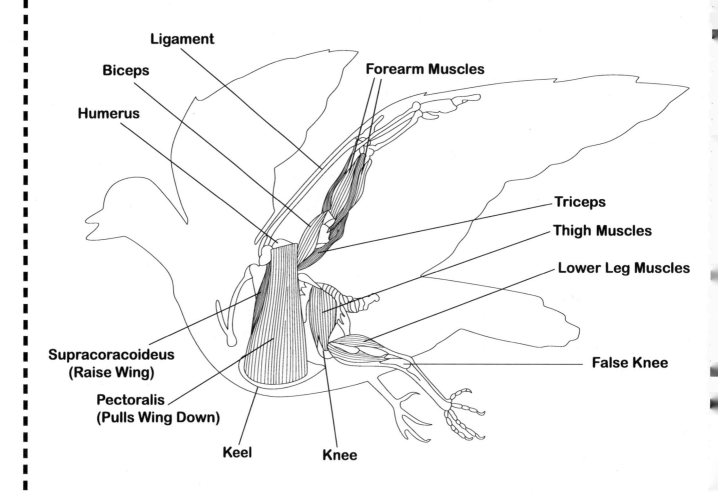

Ligament

Biceps

Humerus

Forearm Muscles

Triceps

Thigh Muscles

Lower Leg Muscles

Supracoracoideus
(Raise Wing)

Pectoralis
(Pulls Wing Down)

False Knee

Keel

Knee

Internal Organs of Elephant

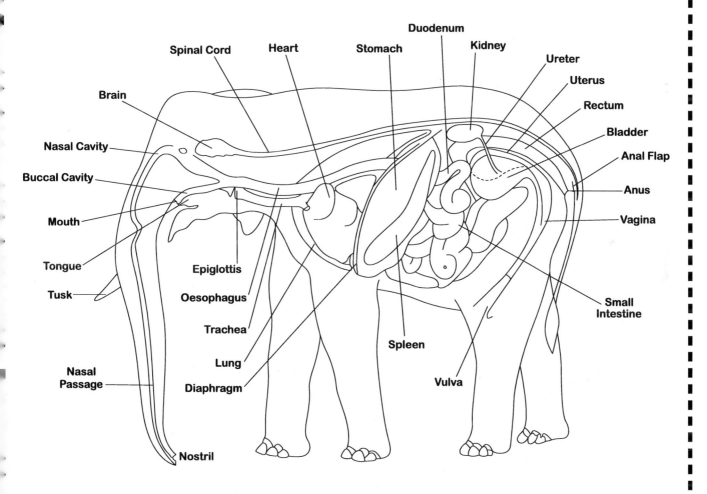

Bones of Elephant

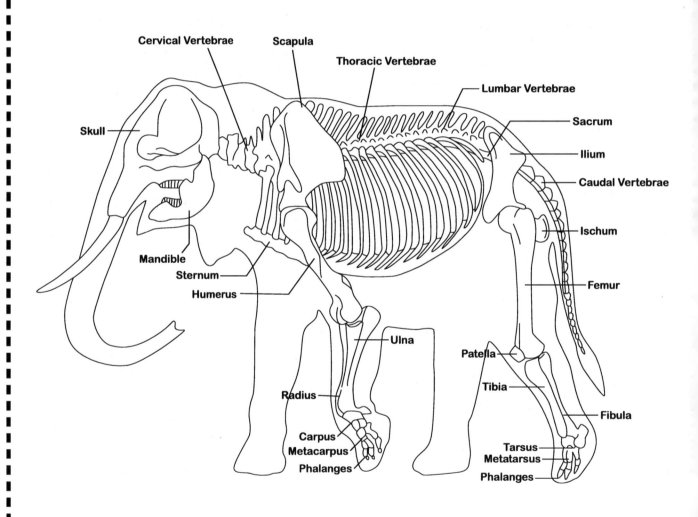

Muscles of Elephant

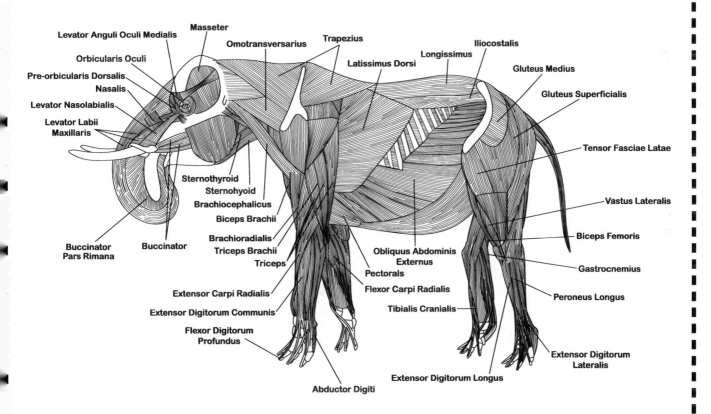

Levator Anguli Oculi Medialis
Masseter
Omotransversarius
Trapezius
Iliocostalis
Longissimus
Latissimus Dorsi
Gluteus Medius
Orbicularis Oculi
Gluteus Superficialis
Pre-orbicularis Dorsalis
Nasalis
Levator Nasolabialis
Levator Labii Maxillaris
Tensor Fasciae Latae
Sternothyroid
Sternohyoid
Brachiocephalicus
Biceps Brachii
Vastus Lateralis
Brachioradialis
Triceps Brachii
Biceps Femoris
Buccinator Pars Rimana
Buccinator
Triceps
Obliquus Abdominis Externus
Gastrocnemius
Pectorals
Extensor Carpi Radialis
Flexor Carpi Radialis
Peroneus Longus
Extensor Digitorum Communis
Tibialis Cranialis
Flexor Digitorum Profundus
Extensor Digitorum Lateralis
Abductor Digiti
Extensor Digitorum Longus

Internal Organs of Dolphin

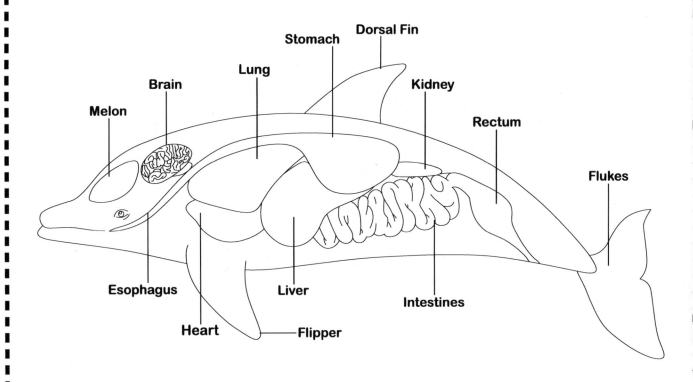

Bones of Dolphin

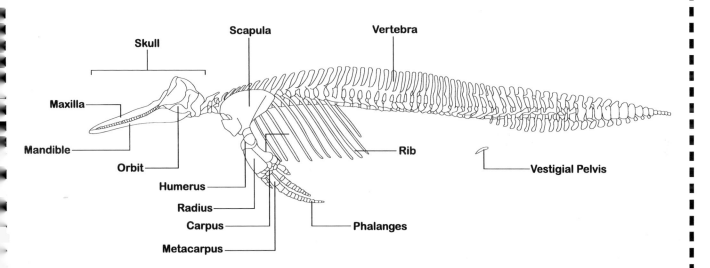

Muscles of Dolphin

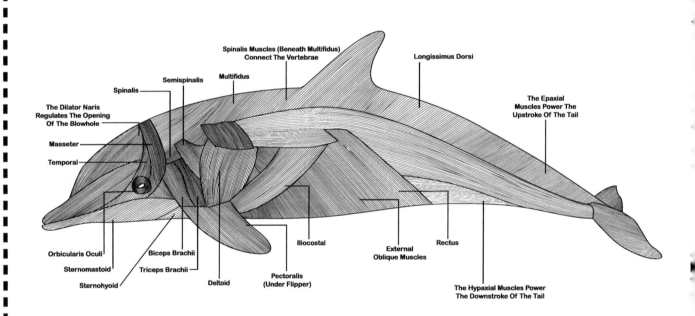

Internal Organs of Deer

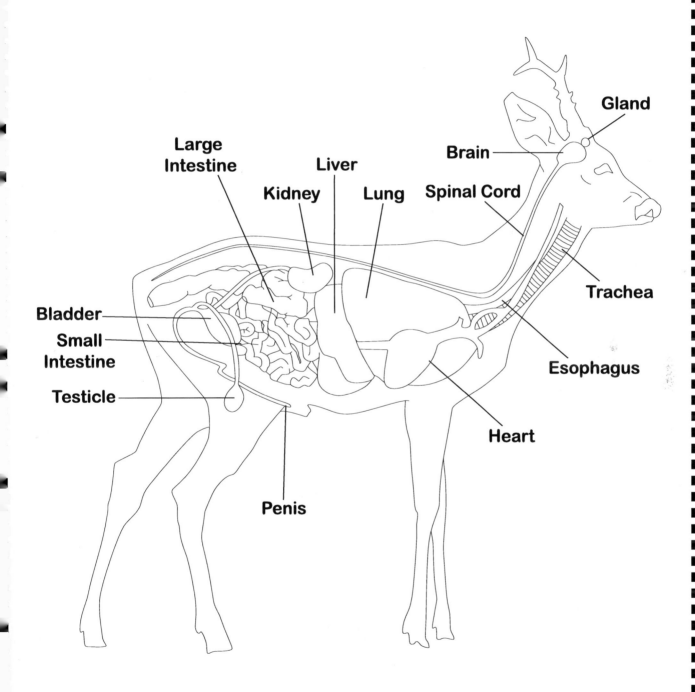

Bones of Deer

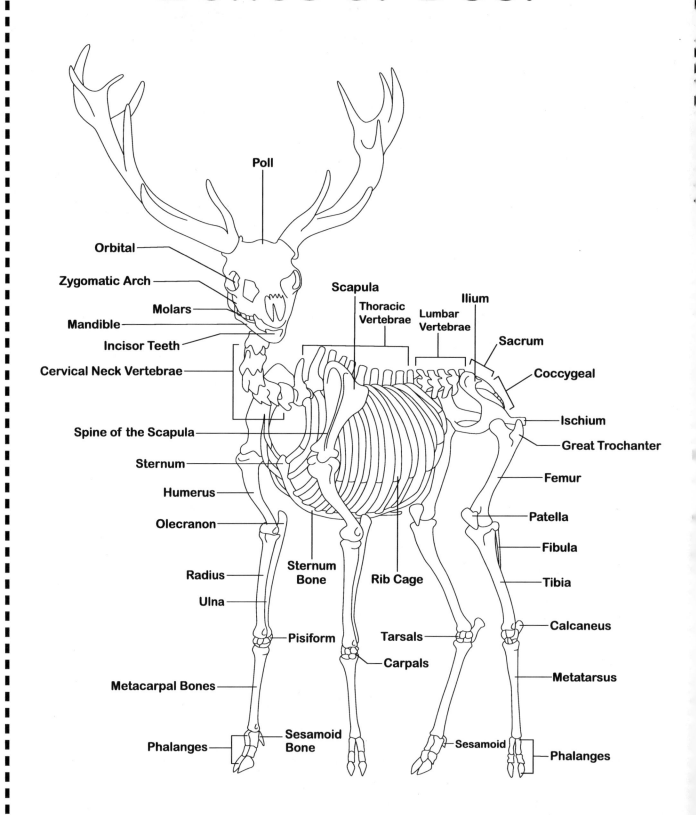

Poll

Orbital

Zygomatic Arch

Molars

Mandible

Incisor Teeth

Cervical Neck Vertebrae

Spine of the Scapula

Sternum

Humerus

Olecranon

Radius

Ulna

Pisiform

Metacarpal Bones

Phalanges

Sternum Bone

Sesamoid Bone

Scapula

Thoracic Vertebrae

Lumbar Vertebrae

Ilium

Sacrum

Rib Cage

Tarsals

Carpals

Coccygeal

Ischium

Great Trochanter

Femur

Patella

Fibula

Tibia

Calcaneus

Metatarsus

Sesamoid

Phalanges

Muscles of Deer

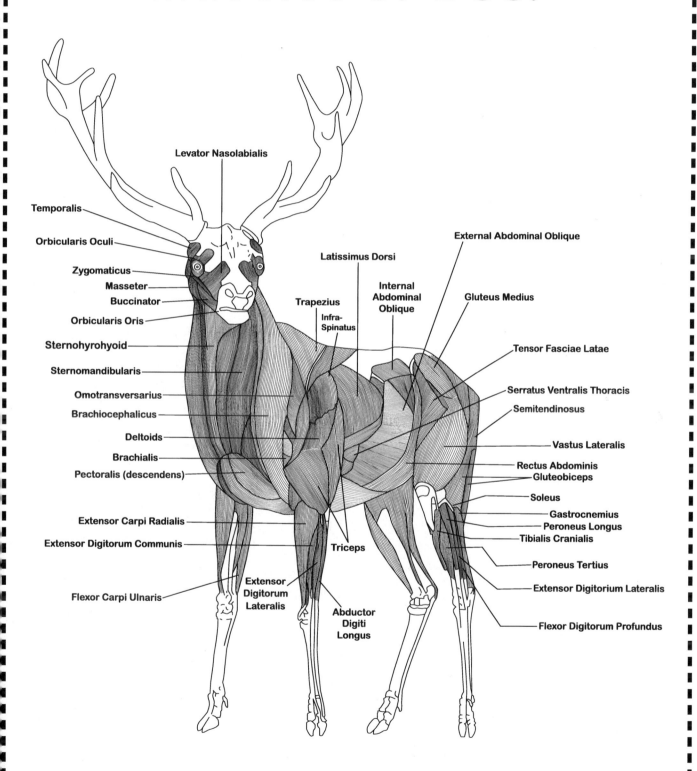

Levator Nasolabialis

Temporalis

Orbicularis Oculi

Zygomaticus

Masseter

Buccinator

Orbicularis Oris

Sternohyrohyoid

Sternomandibularis

Omotransversarius

Brachiocephalicus

Deltoids

Brachialis

Pectoralis (descendens)

Extensor Carpi Radialis

Extensor Digitorum Communis

Flexor Carpi Ulnaris

Extensor Digitorum Lateralis

Abductor Digiti Longus

Triceps

Latissimus Dorsi

Trapezius

Infra-Spinatus

Internal Abdominal Oblique

External Abdominal Oblique

Gluteus Medius

Tensor Fasciae Latae

Serratus Ventralis Thoracis

Semitendinosus

Vastus Lateralis

Rectus Abdominis

Gluteobiceps

Soleus

Gastrocnemius

Peroneus Longus

Tibialis Cranialis

Peroneus Tertius

Extensor Digitorium Lateralis

Flexor Digitorum Profundus

Internal Organs of Zebra

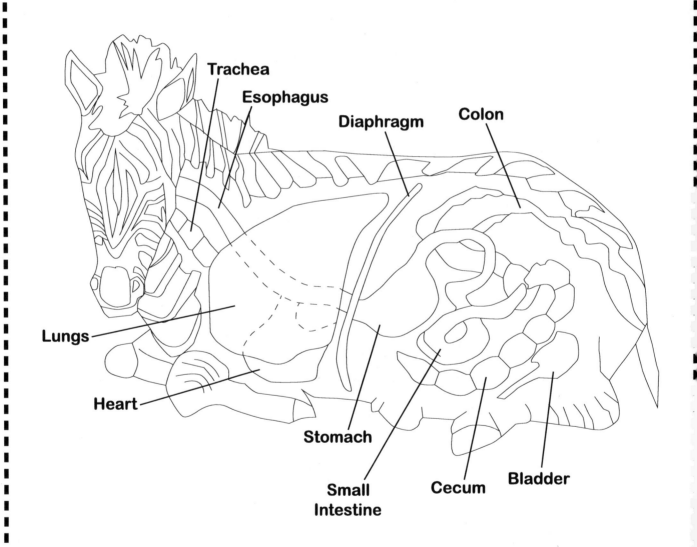

Bones of Zebra

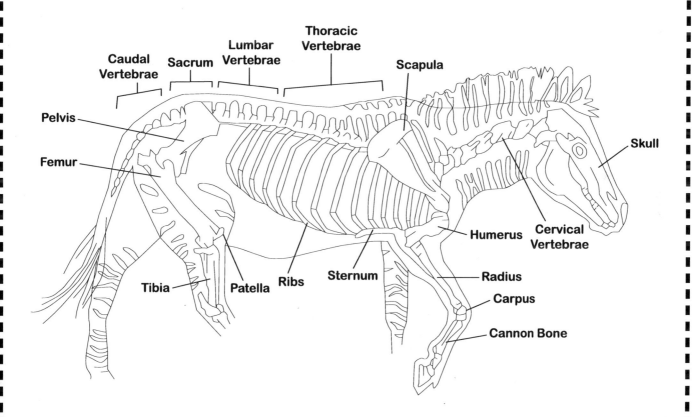

Muscles of Zebra

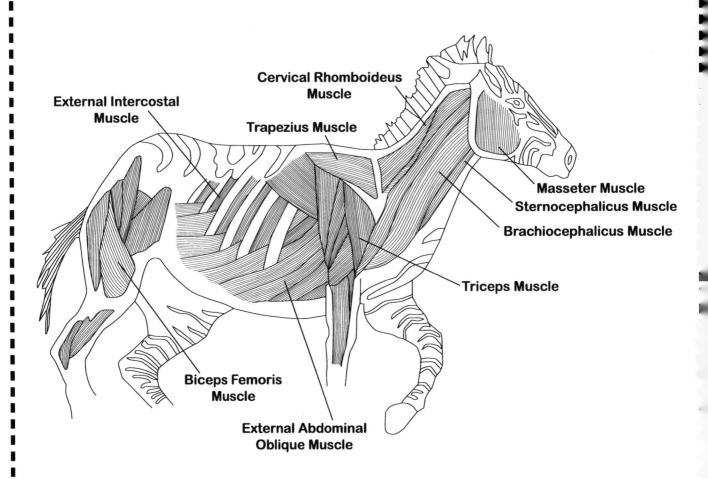

External Intercostal
Muscle

Cervical Rhomboideus
Muscle

Trapezius Muscle

Masseter Muscle

Sternocephalicus Muscle

Brachiocephalicus Muscle

Triceps Muscle

Biceps Femoris
Muscle

External Abdominal
Oblique Muscle

Internal Organs of Tiger

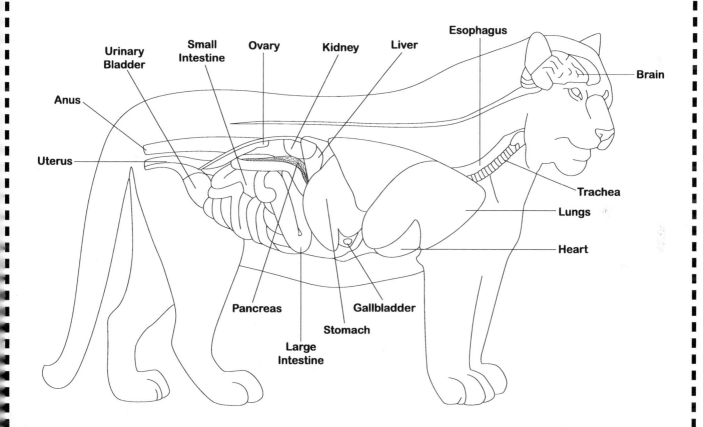

Bones of Tiger

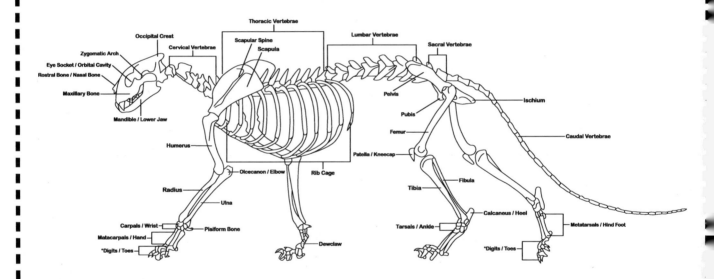

Muscles of Tiger

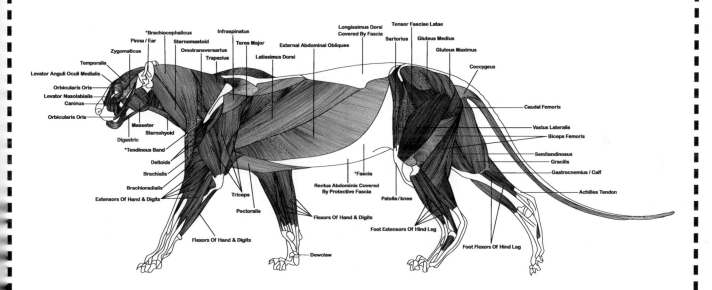

Bones of Bear

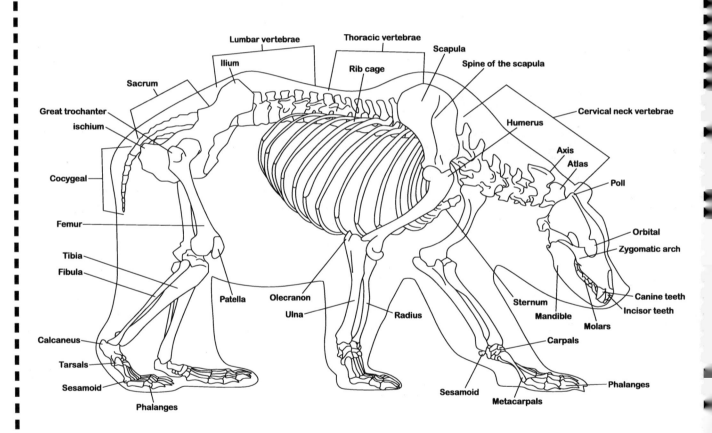

Muscles of Bear

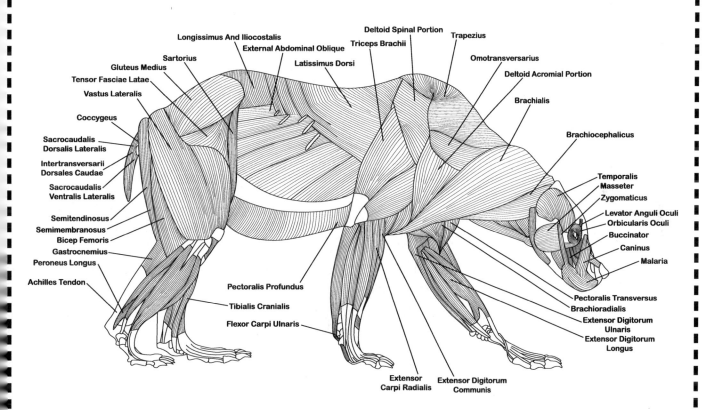

Longissimus And Iliocostalis
External Abdominal Oblique
Sartorius
Gluteus Medius
Latissimus Dorsi
Tensor Fasciae Latae
Vastus Lateralis
Coccygeus
Sacrocaudalis
Dorsalis Lateralis
Intertransversarii
Dorsales Caudae
Sacrocaudalis
Ventralis Lateralis
Semitendinosus
Semimembranosus
Bicep Femoris
Gastrocnemius
Peroneus Longus
Achilles Tendon
Deltoid Spinal Portion
Triceps Brachii
Trapezius
Omotransversarius
Deltoid Acromial Portion
Brachialis
Brachiocephalicus
Temporalis
Masseter
Zygomaticus
Levator Anguli Oculi
Orbicularis Oculi
Buccinator
Caninus
Malaria
Pectoralis Transversus
Brachioradialis
Extensor Digitorum
Ulnaris
Extensor Digitorum
Longus
Pectoralis Profundus
Tibialis Cranialis
Flexor Carpi Ulnaris
Extensor
Carpi Radialis
Extensor Digitorum
Communis

Bones of Hippo

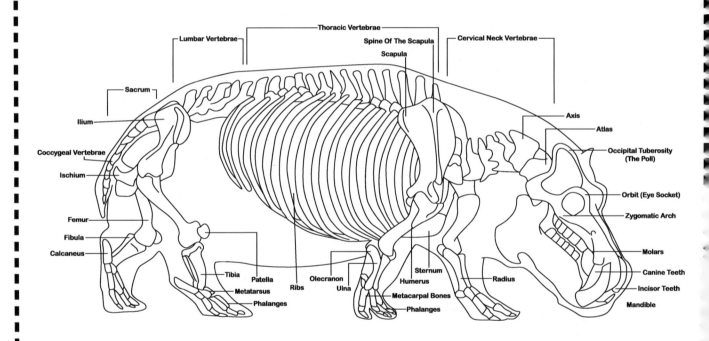

Muscles of Hippo

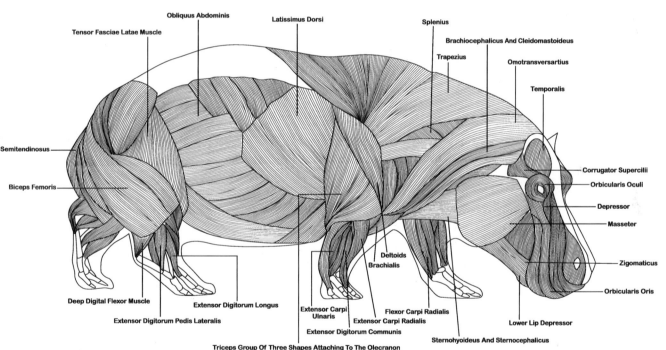

Tensor Fasciae Latae Muscle

Obliquus Abdominis

Latissimus Dorsi

Splenius

Brachiocephalicus And Cleidomastoideus

Trapezius

Omotransversartius

Temporalis

Semitendinosus

Corrugator Supercilii

Orbicularis Oculi

Biceps Femoris

Depressor

Masseter

Deltoids

Brachialis

Zigomaticus

Orbicularis Oris

Deep Digital Flexor Muscle

Extensor Digitorum Longus

Extensor Carpi Ulnaris

Flexor Carpi Radialis

Extensor Digitorum Pedis Lateralis

Extensor Carpi Radialis

Lower Lip Depressor

Extensor Digitorum Communis

Sternohyoideus And Sternocephalicus

Triceps Group Of Three Shapes Attaching To The Olecranon

Bones of Rhinoceros

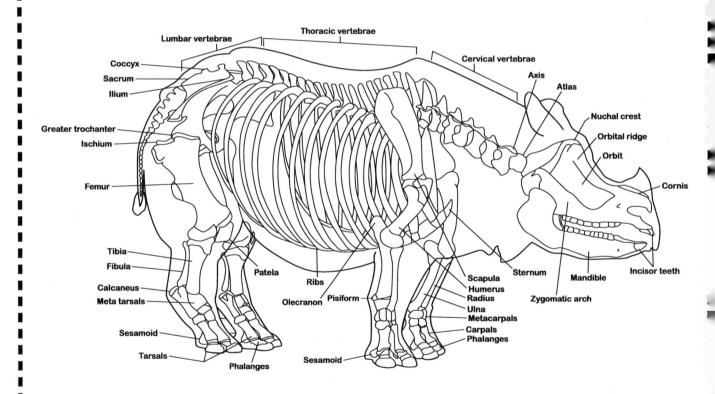

Muscles of Rhinoceros

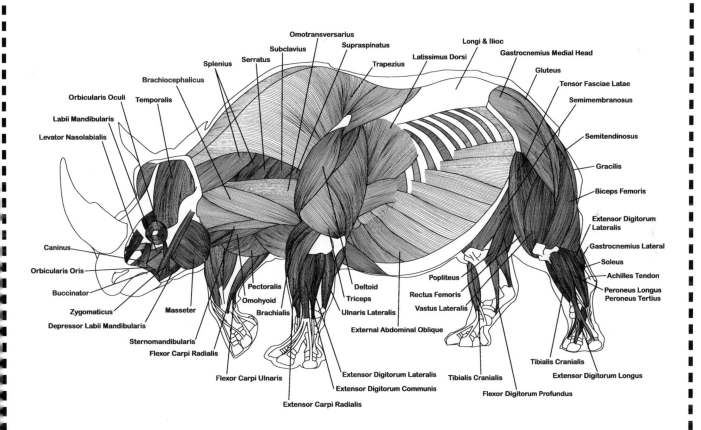

Bones of Wolf

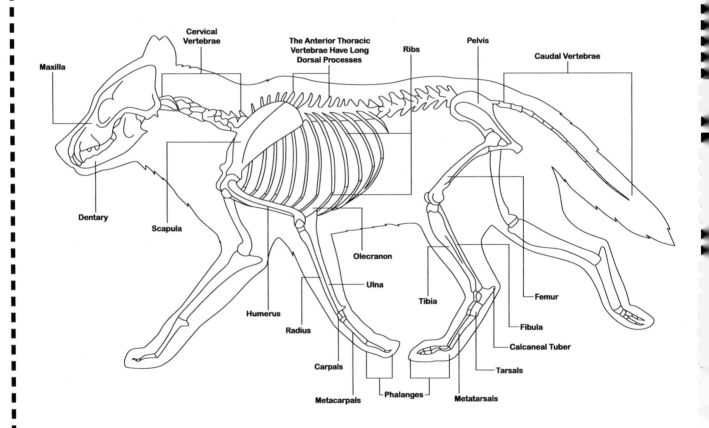

Maxilla

Cervical
Vertebrae

The Anterior Thoracic
Vertebrae Have Long
Dorsal Processes

Ribs

Pelvis

Caudal Vertebrae

Dentary

Scapula

Olecranon

Ulna

Tibia

Femur

Humerus

Radius

Fibula

Calcaneal Tuber

Carpals

Tarsals

Metacarpals

Phalanges

Metatarsals

Muscles of Wolf

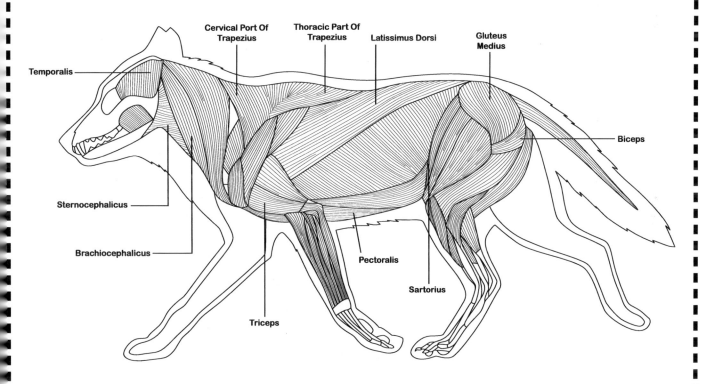

Cervical Port Of Trapezius

Thoracic Part Of Trapezius

Latissimus Dorsi

Gluteus Medius

Temporalis

Biceps

Sternocephalicus

Brachiocephalicus

Pectoralis

Sartorius

Triceps

Bones of Giraffe

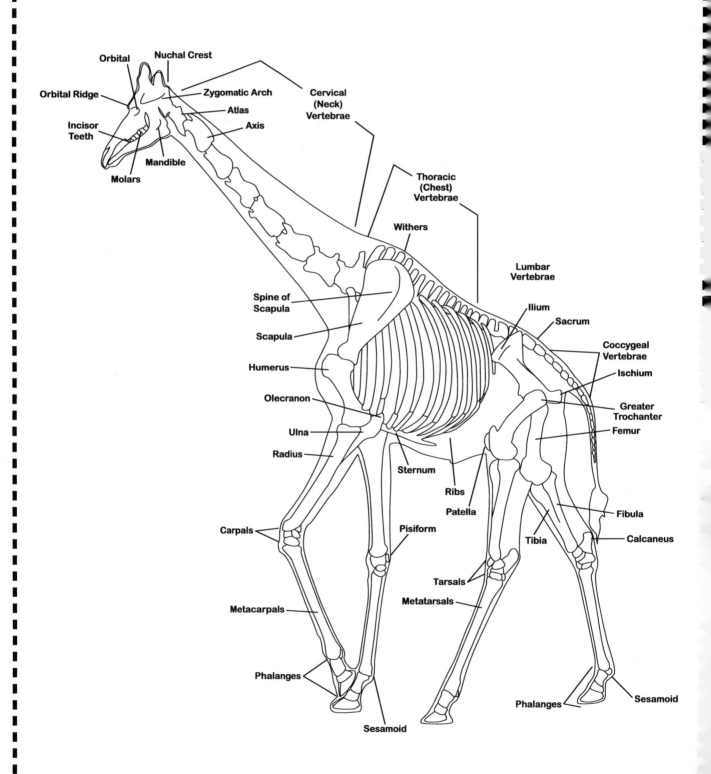

Muscles of Giraffe

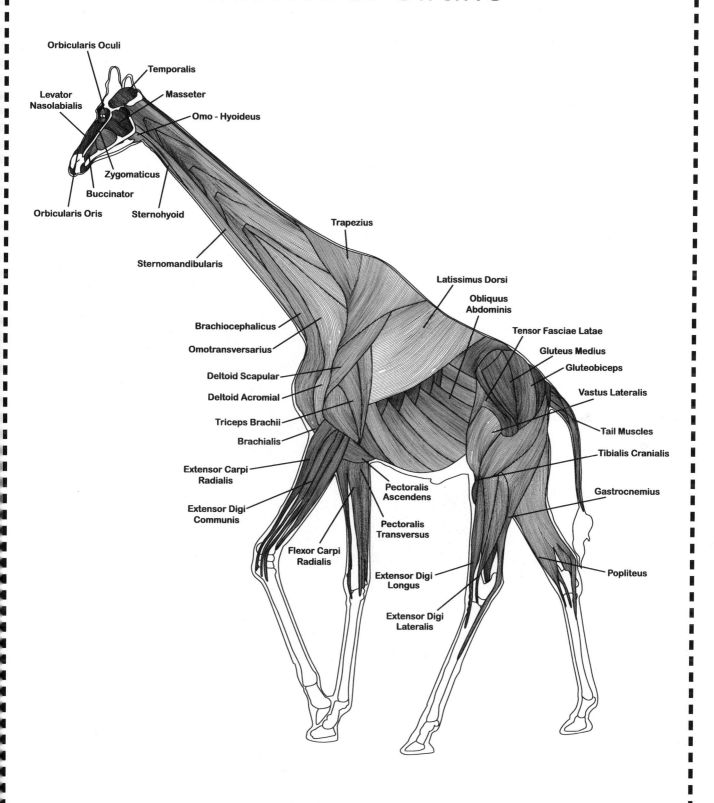

Bones of Camel

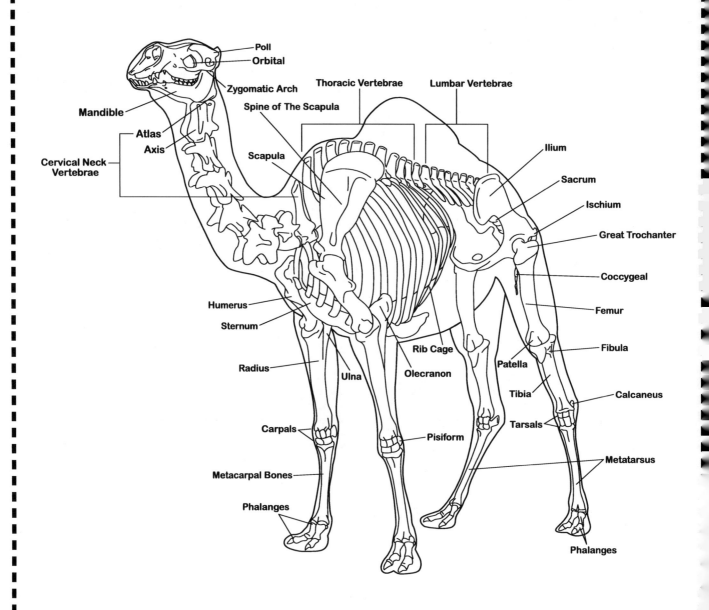

Muscles of Camel

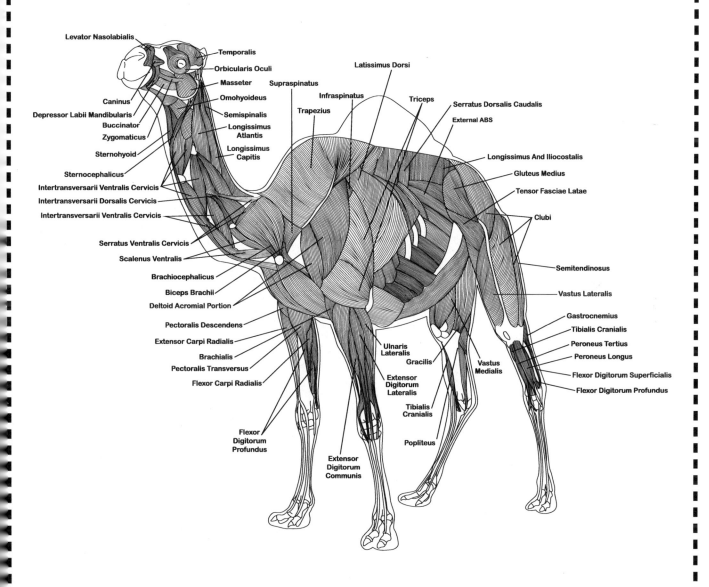

Levator Nasolabialis
Temporalis
Orbicularis Oculi
Masseter
Supraspinatus
Latissimus Dorsi
Caninus
Omohyoideus
Infraspinatus
Triceps
Depressor Labii Mandibularis
Semispinalis
Trapezius
Serratus Dorsalis Caudalis
Buccinator
Longissimus Atlantis
External ABS
Zygomaticus
Sternohyoid
Longissimus Capitis
Sternocephalicus
Longissimus And Iliocostalis
Intertransversarii Ventralis Cervicis
Gluteus Medius
Intertransversarii Dorsalis Cervicis
Tensor Fasciae Latae
Intertransversarii Ventralis Cervicis
Clubi
Serratus Ventralis Cervicis
Scalenus Ventralis
Semitendinosus
Brachiocephalicus
Vastus Lateralis
Biceps Brachii
Deltoid Acromial Portion
Gastrocnemius
Pectoralis Descendens
Tibialis Cranialis
Extensor Carpi Radialis
Peroneus Tertius
Brachialis
Ulnaris Lateralis
Peroneus Longus
Pectoralis Transversus
Gracilis
Vastus Medialis
Flexor Digitorum Superficialis
Flexor Carpi Radialis
Extensor Digitorum Lateralis
Flexor Digitorum Profundus
Tibialis Cranialis
Flexor Digitorum Profundus
Extensor Digitorum Communis
Popliteus

Bones of Mountain Lion

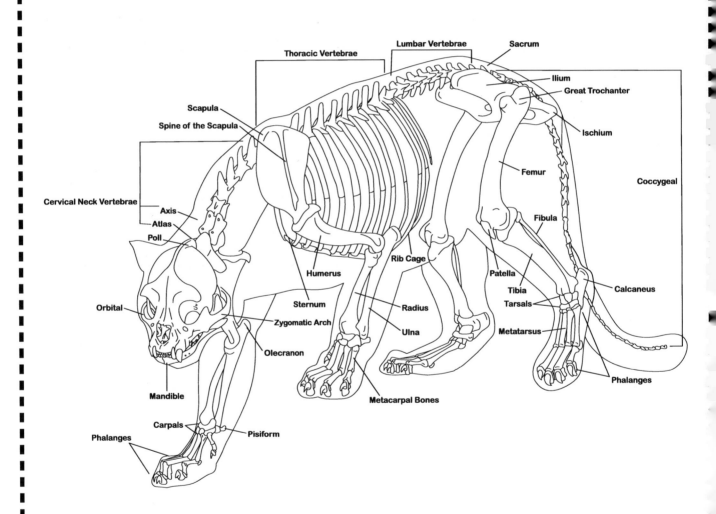

Muscles of Mountain Lion

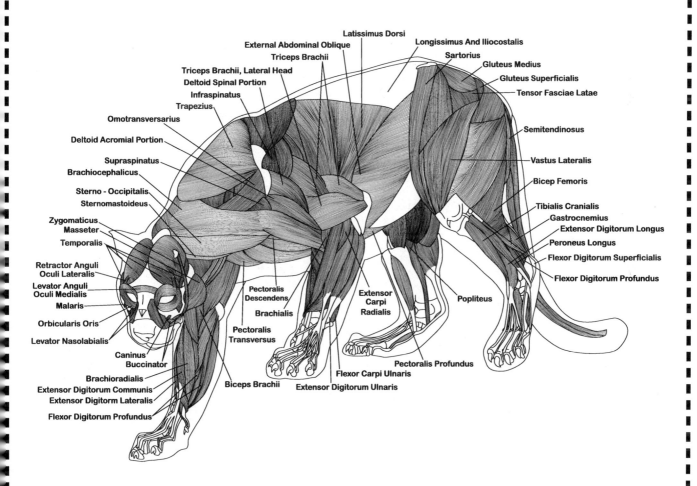

Bones of Red Kangaroo

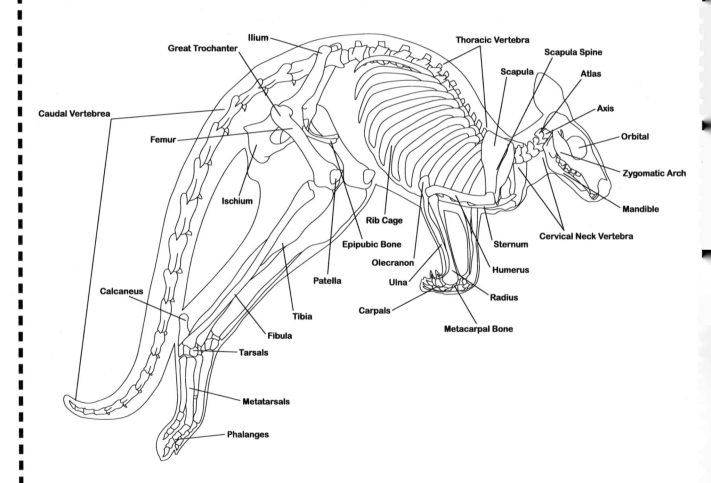

Muscles of Red Kangaroo

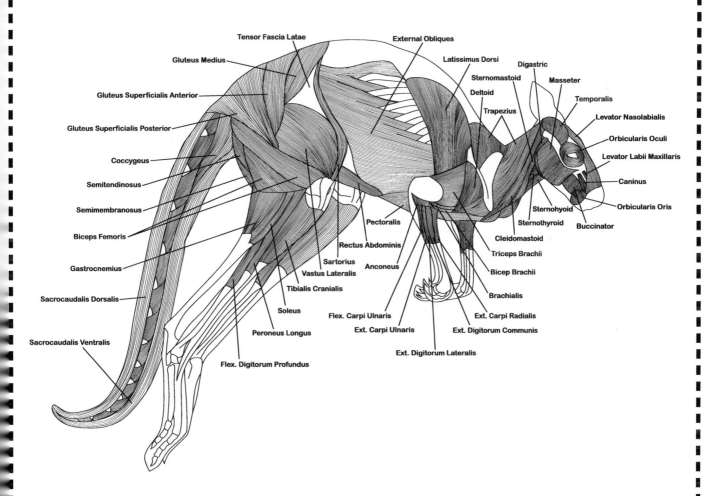

Bones of Jack Rabbit

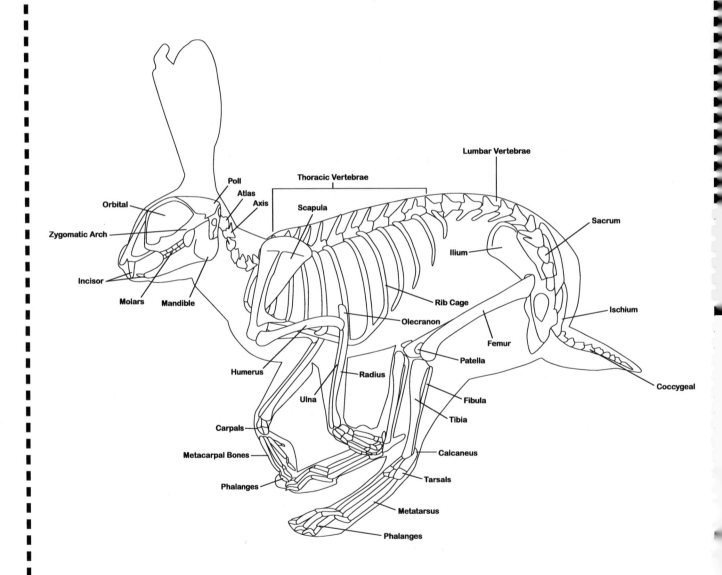

Muscles of Jack Rabbit

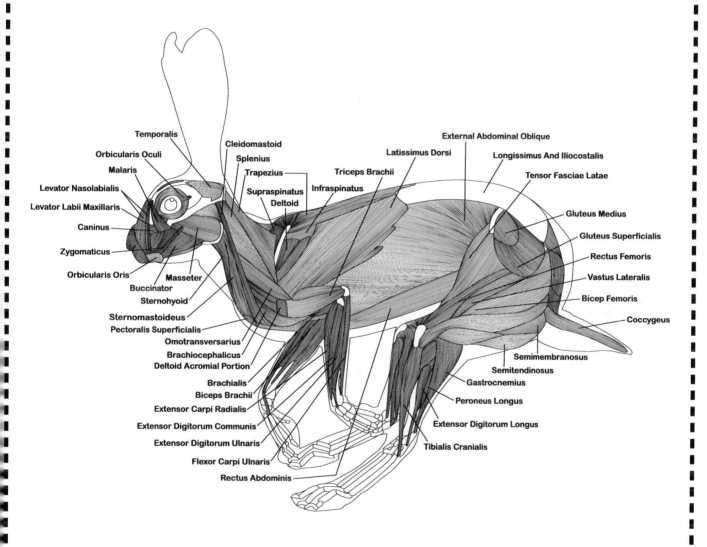

Temporalis
Orbicularis Oculi
Malaris
Levator Nasolabialis
Levator Labii Maxillaris
Caninus
Zygomaticus
Orbicularis Oris
Masseter
Buccinator
Sternohyoid
Sternomastoideus
Pectoralis Superficialis
Omotransversarius
Brachiocephalicus
Deltoid Acromial Portion
Brachialis
Biceps Brachii
Extensor Carpi Radialis
Extensor Digitorum Communis
Extensor Digitorum Ulnaris
Flexor Carpi Ulnaris
Rectus Abdominis

Cleidomastoid
Splenius
Trapezius
Supraspinatus
Deltoid

Triceps Brachii
Infraspinatus

Latissimus Dorsi

External Abdominal Oblique
Longissimus And Iliocostalis
Tensor Fasciae Latae
Gluteus Medius
Gluteus Superficialis
Rectus Femoris
Vastus Lateralis
Bicep Femoris
Coccygeus
Semimembranosus
Semitendinosus
Gastrocnemius
Peroneus Longus
Extensor Digitorum Longus
Tibialis Cranialis

Internal Organs of Guinea Hen

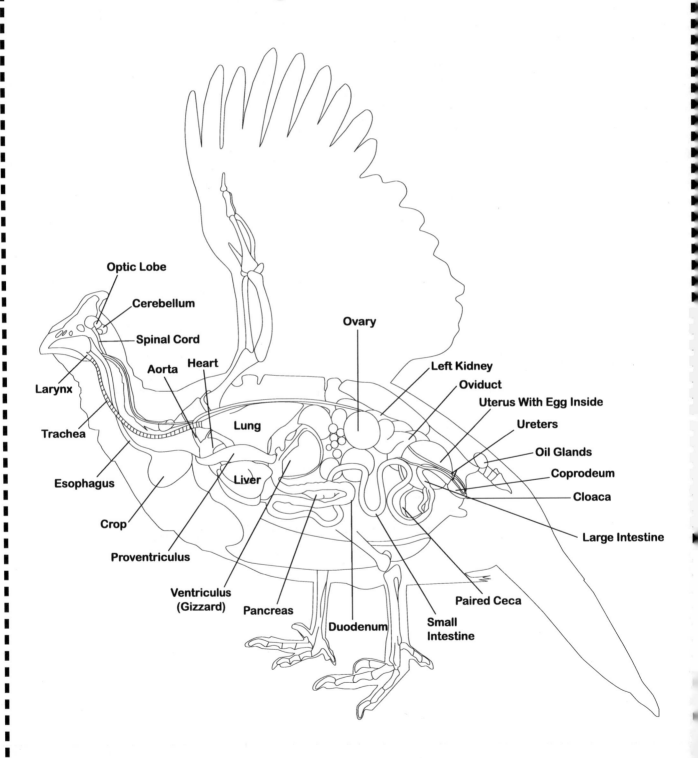

Muscles of Guinea Hen

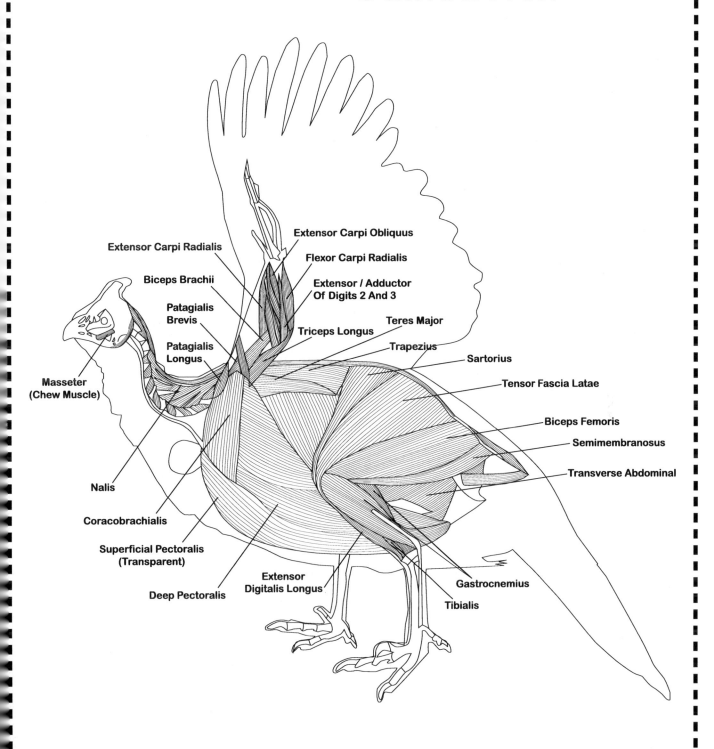

Internal Organs of Chicken

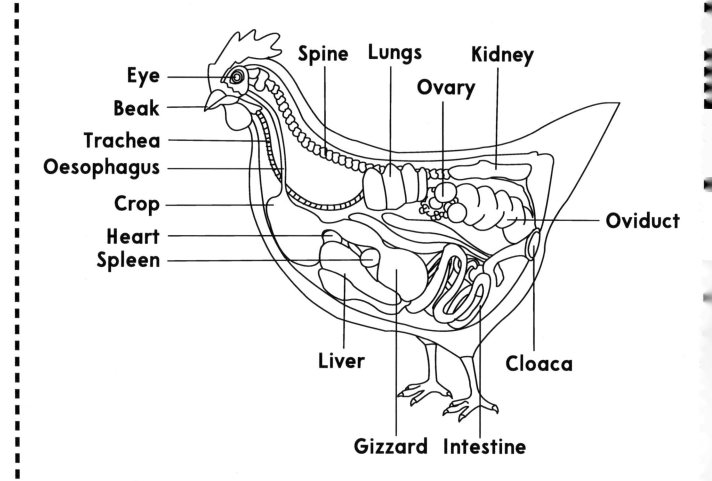

Bones of Chicken

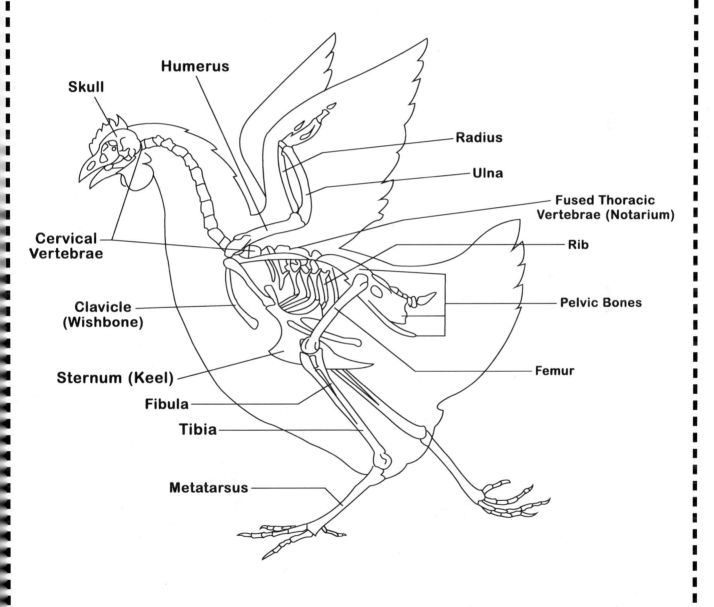

Skull

Humerus

Radius

Ulna

Fused Thoracic
Vertebrae (Notarium)

Rib

Cervical
Vertebrae

Pelvic Bones

Clavicle
(Wishbone)

Femur

Sternum (Keel)

Fibula

Tibia

Metatarsus

Thank You

Made in the USA
Las Vegas, NV
26 November 2024

12742958R00037